Why Chronic Lyme Doesn't
(And Does)
Exist

Finding Common Ground In The Lyme Wars

Dr. Christopher Maloney, N.D.

DEDICATION

To my patients, you have taught me so much. I value you all.

CONTENTS

ACKNOWLEDGMENTS

I want to thank Swarthmore College for helping me think, Harvard University for giving me my pre-medical diploma, and NUNM for giving me a medical degree. Then I started my true education and learned everything about being a doctor from my patients. Thank you, my patients, for reading through the book and letting me know how it could be better.

PREFACE

We're concerned about Lyme disease. It has now been reported globally, and in the U.S. the cases of Lyme have increased nine-fold since reporting started in 1982.[i] We want answers. What is it? How can I avoid getting it? How bad is it? What do I do to keep myself safe?

But we don't have clear answers. Instead, you hear different things from different people. A family member is talking about Chronic Lyme, but your doctor says it doesn't exist. Who's right? Why can't you just get the truth about Lyme?

There's a war going on. The victims of the war are people like you, people concerned about Lyme disease. And regardless of who you talk to about Lyme, chances are good that you're being told one side of the story. The Lyme Wars have taken on religious levels of faith, with both sides claiming absolute truth and heaping scorn on their opponents, the unbelievers.

As you may have guessed, I'm a heretic. I don't believe either side. Not because both don't have good, medical evidence to support their views, but because both have abandoned any middle ground.

It's rare to write a book that I know will upset my colleagues on both sides of the Lyme Wars. But I need to write it for you, the patients. My colleagues on either side will forgive me, for we are all sworn to protect our patients' best interests.

In this book I want to explain the history and arguments of the Lyme Wars, and give you the best medical answers we have about what you should do to keep yourself safe. I also want to lay out the argument that both sides may be right. (Shhh. Listen. That sound you hear, that's the sound of heads exploding in medical offices across the country as my colleagues read these words). Chronic Lyme does and doesn't exist.

We need someone to come to the middle, so that newly diagnosed people understand why they get conflicting information and people who suspect they may have Lyme can learn to navigate their way to health.

If this book keeps one patient from getting unnecessary IV antibiotics, or helps one patient get needed antibiotics even though her doctor said she didn't have Lyme, then it will be time well spent. I'm willing to upset the true believers and the faithful on both sides of the Lyme Wars to help the victims get the help they need.

1 The B.L.T. (Before Lyme's Time) Era

Once upon a time, there was a disease called erythema chronica migrans (ECM). Oh, I know, you came here for Lyme disease. We're talking about the same thing, before it was called Lyme. Think of it as the calm before the storm.

While both sides of the Lyme Wars like to pretend that Lyme suddenly appeared, it's been around for quite a while. Before it was called Lyme, and before the two sides of the Lyme Wars dug themselves into their ideological trenches, doctors had a completely different attitude about the disease.

Before Lyme was Lyme, it was called erythema chronica migrans (ECM), a rare skin disease that responded really well to antibiotics. It only made the dermatological journals, where skin doctors traded tips on how to help their skin patients. They passed on the tip about a weird rash that got better faster with antibiotics. No one seemed very concerned about it.

It wasn't that ECM was extremely rare or harmless. Medical journals report ECM in Sweden back in 1909.[ii] As far back as 1922 German doctors recorded rare brain side effects they associated with the rash.[iii] So it was common, and it occasionally caused severe symptoms long before it was called Lyme.

How old is Lyme really? Researchers now think Ötzi the iceman, who is over five thousand years old, may have had Lyme.[iv] But he probably didn't call it Lyme. He probably called it, "Ugh!" Who knows? Ötzi was murdered, so maybe he was arguing with another shaman about how to treat his Lyme even then.

Back in the good old days before it was called Lyme, a lot of people got bitten by ticks. Most of them were fine. Some of them got a rash that went away with antibiotics. A few of them had severe heart problems from the bites, and a very few of them had serious nerve problems or arthritis as a result of getting bitten. So what changed?

2 Lyme, The War Begins

Something strange happened to Lyme in the summer of 1975.[v]

Cases of ECM had been spreading slowly around the area of Lyme, Connecticut, for a few years. But in 1975 it went nuts. Everyone was getting it. But it wasn't just a rash, because lots of young people and kids were coming down with arthritis symptoms. An entire community was really suffering and wanted answers.

A sudden outbreak of crippling arthritis in children? It made the news. Suddenly we had a new disease. It got called Lyme after the town because no one was sure what caused it. It was a great mystery and it remained a mystery for almost ten years.

The first cases of Lyme started in 1972[vi] and the disease wasn't identified as being caused by the Lyme bacteria, a twisty little spirochete, until 1981. A decade is a long time to have an unknown disease, and people were freaking out. Conspiracy theorists said it was a new military weapon cooked up by the animal lab on Plum Island ten miles away. It had gotten out to kill us all.[vii] Some of the conspiracy theorists still believe that.

Whatever happened to turn ECM into the more aggressive Lyme in the 1970's has continued, with current estimates of Lyme arthritis occurring in 30% of undiagnosed patients.[viii] Or is it 60%?[ix] It's hard to know who's right today since we've got two different sides publishing studies and contradicting each other. Neurological symptoms (brain damage or nerve damage) can occur in 15% of patients.[x] For the non-conspiracy theorists out there, it is possible that Lyme mutated in the 1970's without government help. It may have mutated again recently, because the Mayo Clinic found a new strain.[xi]

The sudden onset of Lyme in the U.S. created many of the conflicts in the Lyme Wars we see today. The first issue was that Lyme was an unknown cluster illness for almost a decade before we knew what caused it. Most cluster illnesses are caused by things like infectious outbreaks or environmental toxins. So the level of fear around cluster outbreaks is at a "pandemic" level rather than a "flu season" level of concern. The medical equivalent of SWAT teams were called in, going over every aspect of the Lyme area. They considered everything from radiation spills to heavy metal poisoning, even after the first lab tests started confirming it was a tick-borne illness.

If the outbreak had been in another state, it might not have created as much of a stir. But the outbreak happened in Connecticut, which has more doctors than you can shake a stick at. These doctors were very concerned about the young patients, many of them children. So the information about the illness got disseminated very quickly. Long before it was confirmed as Lyme, doctors were trying all sorts of treatments. They were battling brain symptoms and severe arthritis. So the local docs were motivated to start some treatment now, rather than waiting for confirmation of what it was before they treated.[xii]

These local doctors were creating treatment plans based on guesswork. If they saw improvements, they continued treatments. It was empirical medicine (observation), not evidence-based (randomized studies) medicine, but seeing is often believing. After months of getting antibiotics, even as long as two years, some patients' symptoms improved. Remember, these treatments were not based on lab testing, because the Lyme lab testing hadn't been invented yet.

After Lyme was identified as the Lyme spirochete in 1981, the local doctors in Connecticut kept doing what had worked for their patients. Some of them found long term antibiotics were helpful with symptoms. They didn't care that large group studies of Lyme patients showed no help from long term antibiotics. These doctors have been treating what they saw as Chronic Lyme cases for decades with some improvement. They were going to ignore larger negative studies because they could point to individual cases within their practices where there was some improvement.

The other problem with the Lyme outbreak in Connecticut was the level of professional personal pride that the local doctors had about their work. In the medical world there is a hierarchy of doctors, with those coming out of the best schools and teaching hospitals getting to tell other doctors they're wrong. But some of the local doctors living around Lyme were the best and the brightest, trained at Yale or affiliated with it. There wasn't anyone that they respected more than one another to tell them they were wrong.

So Lyme presented as an unknown disease within a community of highly intelligent and skilled doctors. The delay in finding a cause gave them a decade to experiment with what might work before the disease was identified as the Lyme spirochete. They'd been healing patients for a decade without knowing what it was they were healing. So when other doctors didn't find benefit from their treatments and told them to stop, they resisted. Especially since those telling them to stop didn't have any new treatments to try.

The locally-treating doctors asked the other doctors about how to care for the patients. What were they supposed to do? To which the official response was basically, "We don't know what to do with those patients, but we don't think what you're doing is going to work. So just leave them alone until we figure out a new treatment."

Of course some of the locally-treating doctors ignored this advice and kept trying, setting up the current Lyme Wars. It's a battle within modern medicine between top-of-the-line smart MDs on both sides who fundamentally don't agree about how to treat Lyme.

3 The CDC (a.k.a., The Villain)

If you read anything about the Lyme Wars online, the part of the villain is often played by the Centers for Disease Control and Prevention (CDC). According to the other side, the CDC is either willfully ignorant or even conspiring to suppress information about Lyme. Its nefarious purpose must be to refuse necessary care from desperate patients. But none of this may be true.

The CDC has many jobs. One of them is to find out about outbreaks and to help stop them, so the CDC was monitoring the Lyme outbreak in Connecticut from its first announcement. They wanted to find the cause more than anyone.

A second job of the CDC is to calm the public and manage health care recommendations. They focus on minimizing costs and avoiding panic. Testing everyone who wanted to get tested for Lyme disease would be educational, but not a good use of public health care dollars. Asking everyone in the U.S. to get tested for Lyme would give us a sense of how far Lyme has spread, but it would be tremendously expensive and cause public panic.

Along the same line, the CDC has to make an educated guess of who will benefit from antibiotics for Lyme, because we can't just give everyone antibiotics all the time. Well, maybe we could, but it would take a major change in how we funded things (imagine the defense budget being diverted into factories for creating enough antibiotics).

So at the CDC, the goal is to figure out who will benefit most from testing and who will benefit the most from treatment. Nowhere in the CDC's mission statement is the goal, "Give the green light to every single person who wants testing and treatment for Lyme." If that makes them a villain, then sure, they're the bad guys.

Using the best information they had, the CDC made rules (guidelines) about what made a positive test for Lyme. They require two tests. The second, more specific test must show that a person has five positive confirmed genetic markers for Lyme in their blood before they get antibiotics.

Five. Four positive markers for Lyme? No Lyme for you. Five? You've got Lyme. Was the cutoff arbitrary? Probably, but it was the CDC's best estimate of who would benefit from treatment.

More recently, likely from public pressure as much as science, the CDC has agreed to giving everyone who has been bitten by a tick one day of antibiotic. It was a bad compromise, because it satisfied no one.

Adults who have been bitten by a tick and test positive for Lyme (five markers) can get twenty-eight days of antibiotic. So they're happy.

But children, who the CDC worried might have side effects from the preferred antibiotic, used to get a less toxic antibiotic. Now they are given nothing unless they have symptoms. You can imagine this does not go over well with parents.

Again, the CDC has to make guidelines about what constitutes a child. Eight years old? No antibiotic. Nine years old? You're treated like an adult. How many parents have pushed to have little Johnnie bumped up to adult status? (Please, he's eight and three-quarters.)

What about if you still have symptoms after treatment? According to the CDC, all adults ever need is that first round of twenty-eight days of antibiotic to be cured. The whole idea of Lyme going chronic and needing more antibiotics isn't really part of the CDC's worldview.

It's that stance, the absolute refusal to admit that Chronic Lyme is a possibility, that has cost the CDC dearly in the Lyme Wars. In every other area of medicine, doctors learn that absolutes are never absolutes. Even though nine hundred and ninety-nine patients may get completely better under the CDC rules, there's going to be that one patient who just doesn't respond as quickly to antibiotics and needs more than twenty-eight days to get healthy again. Claiming otherwise is silly, and would be laughable except that people are suffering as a result. It's the CDC's refusal to admit any possibility of Chronic Lyme that has kept the Lyme Wars going so long.

But we have to give the CDC credit for being willing to discuss the possibility of Chronic Lyme. The CDC has tried to respond to criticism about dismissing Chronic Lyme by funding several studies giving patients who might have Chronic Lyme more antibiotics. They found no real improvement in the patients overall and there were side-effects from giving patients IV antibiotics.[xiii] Case closed.

So the CDC maintains that Chronic Lyme doesn't exist, calling it Post-Lyme Disease Syndrome, simply to label what many of them think of as a mental condition. But they don't really have a treatment for it, leaving patients to suffer. When there is suffering and no hope of recovery, patients are going to look for anyone else who might offer them hope.

Some doctors have filled that hope gap. They don't agree that Chronic Lyme is a mental condition, pointing out that the symptoms are as bad or worse than other chronic physical illnesses. Even the CDC has to agree with that.[xiv] And these doctors think if you have symptoms, you should try to treat them.

4 ILADS (a.k.a., The Online Good Guys)

If a patient has symptoms from getting bitten but the CDC says they are negative for Lyme most doctors today shrug and tell them they don't have Lyme. But some doctors try the antibiotics anyway, and in some patients those antibiotics work to improve the symptoms. Not surprisingly, many of the doctors doing longer antibiotic treatments are in Connecticut. But now the group has expanded internationally.

Back before they knew what caused Lyme, tales of patient treatment successes started filtering out to other doctors outside Connecticut. Some of those doctors also gave antibiotics, and some also had success. That group of doctors started sharing what worked and what didn't, and eventually they formed the International Lyme and Associated Diseases Society (ILADS).

ILADS is alive and well. They maintain a website (ILADS.org) and among the fun facts they share are:

Lyme is everywhere!

It's easy to catch!

It may give you no warning symptoms!

It will be misdiagnosed and mistreated by the majority of doctors!

So go to your ILADS doctor, the only "Lyme Literate" doctor today![xv]

Implying, of course, that everyone else is "Lyme Illiterate," bringing to mind the idea that other medical doctors can't even read. No animosity or insult intended, I'm sure.

In support of their view, ILADS have a listing of seven hundred medical articles, the first three hundred of which support the idea that Lyme can be chronic rather than just acute. A nice review of those studies also exists on pubmed, which is an easier read, but isn't quite as impressive as a long list.[xvi]

To pick one of the supporting studies of Chronic Lyme at random, some skin biopsies can show Lyme bacteria in the patient's skin up to ten months after treatment.[xvii] But other CDC studies did not find Lyme in patients' skin biopsies.[xviii] Who's right? Maybe they both are. Older studies found Lyme in the skin for up to ten years after a bite, but only in untreated patients.[xix] So the first two studies might be working with two different groups of patients, one still with symptoms and the other without symptoms. But the Lyme Wars mean that no one is exploring that possibility.

The next couple hundred studies on the ILADS' site support the idea that Chronic Lyme can attack your brain and give you dementia, and the final few studies support the idea that you can give Lyme to your sexual partners. Really light, fun reading (if you happen to like horror stories).

If it feels like you've just entered into a different world with ILADS doctors, you have. Instead of the CDC view of Lyme being a relatively mild bacterial infection that can be cleaned up every single time with a month of antibiotics, Lyme to an ILADS doctor is a shape shifting, lightning fast predator. It is smarter than our best antibiotics, and even when hit with a barrage of multiple drugs it resists all efforts to wipe it out.

Most frighteningly, many ILADS doctors believe that Lyme can never be wiped out of the body, requiring constant vigilance and aggressive retreatment at the first sign of symptoms for the rest of a patient's life. Remember the hope that ILADS doctors offered patients who were told it was all in their heads? That hope can be easily lost when patients face the specter of lifelong chronic illness and bankruptcy from lengthy expensive treatment plans that insurance won't cover because the patients officially don't have Lyme (according to the CDC).

I love ILADS doctors for listening to patients and giving them hope. But they lose me and the middle ground when they tell patients that the disease will last the rest of their lives.

5 IDSA (a.k.a., CDC Enforcers)

Back when Lyme was finally diagnosed as being a Lyme spirochete, the medical community breathed a sigh of relief. But over time the treatment for Lyme started to be different in different areas and with different doctors. Some doctors were using years of antibiotics, which seemed a little extreme to other doctors. But maybe they were right to treat longer.

Then the CDC did a couple of larger studies that showed the extra antibiotics didn't make much difference. But the doctors using years of antibiotics kept right on using them. They formed the group called ILADS and called themselves Lyme Literate.

Other doctors, hearing about the unnecessary and possibly dangerous overuse of antibiotics, got upset with ILADS. They started looking at other causes and saying that most of the people diagnosed as Chronic Lyme weren't really Lyme cases at all.[xx]

A lot of doctors think this way. They're officially represented by the older IDSA (Infectious Disease Society of America) and they wrote the Lyme treatment guidelines that the CDC still uses. Let me apologize right now for the fact that the two sides of the Lyme Wars decided to call themselves ILADS and IDSA. For the sake of acronym sanity, even though they're IDSA, we're going to call them all the CDC's doctors. IDSA wrote the CDC's Lyme guidelines, the official position on Lyme. The IDSA members are the enforcers, the ones who "debunk" Chronic Lyme on news shows and in newspaper columns. So we'll call IDSA docs CDC doctors going forward.

Are CDC doctors objective? The CDC Lyme Guidelines were written back in 2006, and when the CDC was forced to reconsider rewriting the guidelines (by an antitrust lawsuit in 2010) they made absolutely no changes.[xxi] That's some serious commitment to a single point of view.

The CDC guidelines recommend not giving any antibiotics for a tick bite unless the tick is properly identified and has been attached for more than a day. Then, and only then, can patients get a single pill of doxycycline. But only if the person is over eight years old because doxycycline could discolor a younger child's teeth.

It's worth pointing out that right here that the CDC guideline could use an update. The CDC itself disproved any risk to children's teeth from doxycycline in 2013 and updated the information elsewhere on their website, but it hasn't been changed in the Lyme guidelines.[xxii]

Instead, the guidelines still recommend no treatment for children under eight. The under-eight kids used to get amoxicillin, but the guidelines say it isn't necessary because if the child comes down with symptoms they can get doxycycline then. That's right, don't treat your children for Lyme because of an outdated guideline that incorrectly states they might have a drug side effect to their teeth. Here we have victims in the Lyme Wars, kids who have to develop arthritis or nerve symptoms before they can get an antibiotic.

When will a person come down with Lyme according to the CDC guidelines? Always within the first thirty days, so they only need to be monitored for thirty days. When they come down with symptoms, they can get any of a number of antibiotics that will completely cure them. Even those that come down with heart involvement or brain involvement will be cured (with very rare exceptions). Later signs of Lyme (showing up after thirty days) rarely occur and can again be treated successfully with a short course of antibiotics. The CDC guidelines take time to point out that long-term treatment for Chronic Lyme is unproven, dangerous, and not recommended. But, in passing, the CDC does doom a few patients: "Lyme borreliosis may sometimes cause permanent tissue damage for which there is no cure."[xxiii]

6 What Else Could It Be?

Before we move on, it's worthwhile looking at the the CDC's claim that most people who suffer from Chronic Lyme don't have Chronic Lyme at all.[xxiv] Yes, this is based on the belief that Chronic Lyme itself doesn't exist, but it's worth thinking about what else could be causing the symptoms.

The symptoms of Chronic Lyme cover a vast area, one that overlaps with many other illnesses. Since Lyme is on the rise, it receives a lot of media attention. But that doesn't necessarily mean that everyone with those symptoms has Chronic Lyme. We need to remember that other illnesses have been considered much more common than they are today.

Back in the 1980s, everything was caused by candida. People did cleanses, they took antifungals, they did treatments. The candida would go away and come flaring right back if you ate so much as a grape. But candida caused every strange symptom picture that a doctor saw, so some doctors found candida everywhere. Except for those doctors that didn't believe candida happened at all. (Many still don't.) They said it was all in the patient's mind.

Then, starting in the 1990's, we had chronic fatigue. This beauty caused all sorts of problems, and patients struggled with it. Lots of lab tests were done, with inconclusive results. But some doctors treated and specialized in chronic fatigue. They had many aggressive treatments. Except for those doctors who didn't believe in it. They said it was all in the patient's mind.

As we reached the new millennia, we had fibromyalgia. These muscle pains overlapped with chronic fatigue. Some doctors specialized in treating fibromyalgia. Except those doctors who decided that it was mental and that the best thing for patients with fibromyalgia was counseling.

Now we've got Chronic Lyme. Some doctors specialize and treat it. Others say it's all in the patients' minds. But that should come as no surprise, because it happens again and again in medical history. One article traces the societal obsession with popular illnesses back to Brucellosis in the 1930's.

At this point, it's clear that many doctors consider Chronic Lyme a "popular" disease. Even if they think Chronic Lyme could exist, they don't think it's that common. To them, Chronic Lyme is filling the public's need to have a "popular disease."

The idea that "popular" diseases are limited to just a few fringe diseases ignores the reality of drug marketing "manufacturing" new diseases. Are things like heartburn and erectile dysfunction really so terrible that we need millions of prescriptions? And, of course, people who hear about a new disease in the news are going to wonder if they have it when they have unexplained symptoms.

So blaming the populace for "popular" diseases ignores the reality that it is doctors and the medical establishment that make these diseases popular by discussing them a great deal.[xxv] The CDC is its own worst enemy. Every time it starts "debunking" Chronic Lyme it popularizes it because the public assumes if there's so much smoke there must be a fire.

But the message here isn't just that some doctors think you're crazy no matter what you tell them. It's that other doctors tend to jump on the new fad bandwagon every decade and run with it with everything they've got. The same doctors who might have prescribed a candida cleanse in the 1980's are selling a drug cocktail for Lyme today. Patients who hear about Chronic Lyme want to be tested for Lyme and treated if there's any possibility. Who's to say that those patients don't have candida? Or chronic fatigue?[xxvi] Or fibromyalgia? Or another illness? Why is it always Lyme?

Just because Lyme is common now doesn't mean it's

everywhere. And when one lab gives positive results that other labs don't recognize, maybe patients should look for another way to rule out Lyme before taking years of treatment. Or at least reconsider six months into treatment whether it couldn't be something else if you haven't gotten better. It might not be Lyme after all.

7 The Lyme Wars

So we have ILADS vs. the CDC, both with lots of research behind them. Each takes an entirely different view on Chronic Lyme.

To ILADS, Lyme is the most sophisticated disease you've ever seen. It really does seem like it must have been engineered in a military lab. As soon as you add antibiotics, it spores up to protect itself. It sneaks through your cells and can outrun your immune system by traveling upstream in your blood. Long after you think you've beaten it, it decloaks itself. It was hiding inside your cells! You can imagine Lyme as a James Bond supervillain, plotting its revenge and coming up with new, fiendishly clever ways to escape all your efforts to destroy it.

To the CDC, Lyme is a pesky nuisance, like an ant hill or a bumbling burglar in a comedy. This goofy fellow trips himself up by showing you exactly where he got into the body with a huge rash. Most of the time he doesn't do anything, and if he does manage to cause problems you can dispatch him easily with a single round of antibiotics. He's certainly not worth worrying about.

So where does your family doctor stand in the Lyme Wars? Most doctors, unless they say they are ILADS or "Lyme Literate," fall into the CDC camp. They may not specialize in Lyme. When you ask for testing they will send the standard test off to their local lab, which processes it in accordance to CDC guidelines.

Patients going to CDC doctors may be told that they don't have Lyme despite having four positive genetic markers (almost five – close, but no Lyme for you). Most may not have Lyme, but at least a few may be experiencing symptoms from Lyme and wait years before they run into an ILADS doctor who will treat them.

8 But My Lyme Lab Came Back Positive

Isn't there an easy solution to the Lyme Wars? Just look at the lab test. If your lab test says you're positive, then you've got Lyme. Once you've been treated, you can see if the test is positive or not. If the test is negative you no longer have Lyme. Isn't it that simple? No.

Anyone who has had a positive Lyme lab and called for a doctor's appointment may have heard the question, "Which lab?" When they answered their local hospital lab, they got no more questions. But if they answered something else, there might have been a long pause at the other end of the phone as the receptionist wrote down that a CDC lab hadn't been done.

There are many alternative Lyme tests, but one major lab stands out for ILADS doctors. IgenX is the major lab that supports all the "extra" antibiotic treatments ILADS doctors give their patients. It's this lab that is the current target of online medical attacks by the CDC. You can read between the lines when the CDC talks about needing "verified and standardized" testing. Things have gotten downright nasty, with the CDC group publishing a critique of "Chronic Lyme disease."[xxvii] (You know you're in trouble when they put your disease in quotes in a medical journal.)

Almost all the labs in the U.S. test Lyme based on CDC guidelines. Five genetic markers makes you positive; less means you're negative.

But IgenX is different. For them, two or three genetic markers are sufficient to confirm Lyme.[xxviii] IgenX argues that their testing is far more complex, but the end result is that they are declaring far more patients positive for Lyme than the CDC. How many more positive? The CDC has estimated that a "private lab" like IgenX (not named in the article) might find as many as 91% of cases positive, while the CDC would only find 8% positive for Lyme.[xxix] That's why a CDC doctor doesn't trust an "alternative" lab result, and patients with a positive IgenX test will face questions and an underlying skepticism about their diagnoses.

That doesn't mean that IgenX is right or wrong. But it does mean that an IgenX result won't be recognized as positive by a CDC-believing doctor. A patient may have paid for an IgenX test with an ILADS doctor, go to their family doctor with positive result, and be refused treatment. This mystifying result is because the doctor does not believe that the IgenX test is accurate. But it can feel to the patient as if the doctor doesn't believe they have Lyme disease (which, honestly, they probably don't). The lack of belief by their family doctor means that patients cannot get insurance coverage for treatment, making treating Chronic Lyme extremely expensive even if you have insurance.

ILADS doctors swear by IgenX and will use it as the basis of all their treatments. So far so good.

But ILADS doctors don't just want to test for Lyme with IgenX, they want to test for all the "co-infections." These are other, lesser-known bugs that can hitchhike along with Lyme in an infected tick.

The co-infections mean that, even if you come back as negative for Lyme from IgenX, you may still need to be treated for one of these other, less well-known infections.

If patients start to feel that most IgenX labs will be positive for something, they're probably right. Even if IgenX labs come back "inconclusive" for Lyme or a co-infection, ILADS doctors can treat or not depending on their preferences. If a patient has symptoms consistent with Lyme or a co-infection (which is a very broad list) chances are patients will be treated. So some ILADS doctors don't bother to even test anymore.

Fortunately, the treatment for the Lyme co-infections may be the same antibiotic an ILADS practitioner would use for Lyme. Unfortunately, sometimes the co-infection treatment involves three or more antibiotics as well as anti-parasitic medications that are about as toxic as they sound. These treatments may be effective, and the ILADS doctors can point to their own small studies that support aggressive treatment. But we don't know enough about the co-infections to say for sure if aggressive treatment is more curative.

Without any standard lab testing, there's no way to resolve the Lyme Wars. ILADS doctors who get IgenX testing are at least creating a record of how effective different treatments are for different levels of Lyme infection. But no one at the CDC is looking at that information because they don't believe in Chronic Lyme, much less the co-infections.

9 The Facts: Which Side Is Right?

Depending on which side of the Lyme Wars you are on, the patients who are still sick and think they have Chronic Lyme are either: a) mentally ill and just think they have Lyme or b) really have Lyme, which is a superbug resistant to all attempts to wipe it out. No, I don't think either one of these is true. But they are the existing options for those who have Lyme symptoms in the U.S. within our current medical model.

We have two groups of very smart, very dedicated MDs who have been at each other's throats for decades now. Rather that coming to a consensus, these two groups are entrenched and call each other names under their breath. They go to separate conferences and use separate labs.

Both sides can point to individual cases and studies that support their viewpoint. But for a patient with Lyme, this conflict can be tremendously confusing and frustrating. Isn't there some way to cut through all the politics and find objective, evidence-based medical information about Lyme? Yes and no.

To find another expert authority we need to leave the U.S. and look at the world stage. There's a group called the Cochrane Database located in Belgium that compiles the world's medical studies. It has experts review all the studies and come up with an opinion. Cochrane tends to be more conservative, and their opinions would tend to favor the CDC viewpoint, but it's worthwhile looking at what they say about Lyme (the drumroll, please).

Cochrane on Lyme: Yes, taking doxycycline can help.

Using the Cochrane database, we can say that using doxycycline when you get a tick bite will lower your risk of getting Lyme (the risk goes down from 2% to less than 1%). The underlying Cochrane message is that only 2% of those bitten without getting an antibiotic came down with Lyme.[xxx] That's some very good news to those of us who live with tick-infested woods.

Cochrane on Nerve Symptoms: We don't know if lots of antibiotics help untreated "Lyme brains."

Both ILADS and the CDC agree that short-term, untreated Lyme can sometimes cause neurological (brain) issues. The Cochrane database looked at whether or not more antibiotics helped untreated nervous system Lyme. They concluded that: "It is not possible to draw firm conclusions" because the studies done by doctors (on either side of the issue) were so poorly done.[xxxi]

It shouldn't be this way. Untreated Lyme brain symptoms respond to antibiotics and both sides want to use antibiotics. But because of the Lyme Wars, no good studies exist that can tell us what the best length of time is needed to treat effectively.

Cochrane on children: We don't have know the best Lyme treatment for children.

Again, the Cochrane database says: "Data is scarce and with limited quality." They couldn't find any studies that supported giving kids longer doses of antibiotics, but that doesn't mean it won't help, only that the studies haven't been done.[xxxii]

Cochrane on the CDC: The CDC guidelines are not the final word on Lyme.

After looking at six different sets of Lyme guidelines worldwide, the Cochrane Database says: "No statement can be given on quality of content and validity of recommendations" probably because we lack good evidence for how to treat Lyme properly.[xxxiii]

Cochrane on lab testing: We don't know the best way to test for Lyme.

Can we get a verdict from the Cochrane Database on the best way to test for Lyme? Is the CDC right and IgenX wrong? Visa versa? Nope. They didn't find any unbiased studies, and the results were heterogeneous, which means they were all over the map.[xxxiv]

Cochrane on Chronic Lyme: We can't say whether or not Chronic Lyme exists.

OK, we don't know how to treat it, we're not sure how to test for it, and we can't really rely on the guidelines, so does Chronic Lyme exist? Cochrane database says: "patients may experience residual symptoms after treatment with a prevalence of approximately 28 %." But those symptoms may or may not be from Lyme.[xxxv]

That's not conclusive, but it does raise the question about Chronic Lyme being just in a patient's head. A generous assessment of mental illness puts it at about 18% of the population in any given year.[xxxvi] Some of the people experiencing Chronic Lyme, at least 10%, are probably not making it up.

Using the Cochrane Database medical experts, we can conclude pretty much absolutely nothing about Lyme. And it's not because there aren't medical studies. Looking up Chronic Lyme disease (ILADS' preferred name) gives over a thousand medical articles. In comparison, the CDC's preferred term, Post-Lyme Disease Syndrome, has less than a hundred studies. So ILADS is winning the definition part of the Lyme Wars, but that means nothing in terms of what is going to be the best treatment for Lyme.

10 The Wisdom Of Dogs: The Co-infections

One of the most annoying things about the Lyme Wars is that my dog has a better handle on Lyme than we humans do. He can get a blood spot test, one drop of blood tells us if he's positive or negative for Lyme. Then he can get a vaccine, and/or a nasty chemical rub that kills the ticks as soon as they bite him (and shortens his life, but hey, it's a tradeoff). So maybe we humans could learn something from the dogs.

Imagine that tomorrow we somehow resolved the Lyme Wars. One side wins, there's one lab and one treatment for Lyme. (You can fantasize about your favorite side clubbing the other side with baguettes, crying "Who's literate now?")

But we've moved on already. ILADS has moved on from Lyme to work on the co-infections. It's like the battlefield keeps shifting, creating a greater and greater distance between the two sides.

They could agree entirely about Lyme tomorrow but be no closer to agreeing about the necessary treatments for the co-infections.

So what do we know about co-infections?

What does the CDC say? Pretty much they don't exist. There's no recommendation to test for them, and no acknowledgement that they co-exist along with Lyme as tick-borne illnesses. Buried at the bottom of the current CDC Lyme guidelines there is a short section that recommends a separate treatment for Babesia, one of the co-infections. But that information is not mentioned in the summary of the Lyme guidelines that most doctors read. When the CDC discusses Lyme testing, there is no CDC recommendation that the labs test for Babesia at the same time.

But within ILADS, co-infections are the focus of what they're treating now. Forget just testing for Lyme, now we're treating this or that newer co-infectious agent (relapsing fever is the infection-of-the-month this year), pushing the limits of what patients will endure in terms of the quantities of drugs they can take.

The cycle of Chronic Lyme treatment in ILADS today is to test using IgenX, treat with a cocktail of multiple drugs, and then retest. Sometimes the treatment works, the Lyme markers fall, and the patient feels better. Sometimes the treatment works, the Lyme markers fall, and the patient feels no different or even worse. At the same time, some Lyme patients continue to have symptoms despite the most aggressive treatment. They currently must choose either ILADS doctors who will continue to test and treat aggressively or CDC doctors who will say it's in their heads. In the extraordinary case where a patient is truly free-and-clear of all Lyme, the reality is that many of them live in a tick and Lyme endemic area. Unless they move to the arctic, they will likely be re-exposed and re-infected. So the entire journey can start all over again. And that's just Lyme, not including all the co-infections.

Usually if a person has improved Lyme markers but continues to have symptoms, ILADers will test for another possible co-infection, but there are always new possible co-infections we can't even test for yet. There is literally no point at which a patient can be declared free-and-clear of any possible recurrence. The rest of a patient's life can be spent getting tested.

So just how common are the co-infections? They include Anaplasmosis, Babesiosis, Bartonellosis, and Erlichiosis. We don't have good information on the spread of these diseases in humans in the U.S. But we do among man's best friend, who evidently got the better health care coverage. U.S. tracking of dogs estimates that more than one in ten dogs with Lyme also have a co-infection.[xxxvii]

While these co-infections would officially only be found in the same tick areas as Lyme, researchers checking dogs in the Caribbean (generally thought to be a Lyme clear zone) found that some of the dogs were infected with Lyme or the other co-infections.

Unlike people, the researchers were able to experiment on the dogs to find out some important information about how Lyme and other co-infections spread. Remember these are dogs, not people. But what happened to the dogs might be relevant to figuring out what happens in people exposed to Lyme.

Only about one in four dogs showed any symptoms from Lyme or the co-infections, but all of them continued to be infections even after treatment with doxycycline.[xxxviii] That's right, treating them didn't make them less infectious.

More importantly, newly infected dogs who were treated had negative labs after they were treated. They were cured according to their lab results.

Dogs who'd had the infection for a while stayed positive for the infection after treatment. According to their labs, they still had Chronic Lyme.

But BOTH sets of dogs, the recently-infected lab-negative "cured" dogs and the lab-positive "Chronic Lyme" dogs, were able to pass the Lyme infection on to ticks that bit them. All these dogs were carriers after treatment, even when their labs said they were clean.

But was it an ongoing infection, or does Lyme just live on at a low grade level in all dogs? Adding a second drug (rifampin) to the treatment did lower the number of dogs who were infectious afterward. So some kind of infectious level continued, even when the labs came back negative.

Any medical researcher who wanted to argue about the relevance of this study would start with the fact that these are dogs. But maybe the lessons of the study can be broadly applied. Most of the infected dogs showed no symptoms, the labs didn't tell you if the dog still had the illness, and most of the dogs stayed as symptom-free carriers of the Lyme. Oh, and Lyme is endemic in areas that the CDC claims it doesn't exist.[xxxix]

Yes, a CDC doctor would reply. But these are dogs. Do you have any proof that human Lyme exists on the Caribbean islands? Yes. A recent report of new human cases found that two-thirds of islanders with rashes were now positive for Lyme.[xl] So the dogs are passing it on to people, or the other way around, despite lacking any of the "right" kind of tick in the area to pass it on.

But we may not even need any animal carriers to be at risk of getting a co-infection. In China a patient with a co-infection managed to infect other patients with her breath. The Chinese hospital documented that the majority of other infected patients had no physical contact with the patient. She did have blood in her mouth, so it may have been blood droplets in the air rather than her saliva alone that spread the infection. But it makes the co-infections almost impossible to avoid.[xli]

The co-infection passed by the Chinese patient was Anaplasmosis, so it may be wise to look at how we test for Anaplasma in the body. While it receives a lot less press than Lyme, Anaplasma has been known for decades for causing "tick-borne" fever that can blow over with no symptoms or be fatal. Because we don't have great tests for Anaplasma, if you don't know what you're looking for you can miss it entirely. You have to test for it specifically and the test isn't that accurate. We don't know how well it travels, its preferred hosts, how fast it can spread. Experts assume it is much more common than it is reported to be.[xlii]

If you suddenly find yourself more frightened by the co-infections than Lyme itself, welcome to the club. Much of the current battle over Chronic Lyme treatment may really be from the mixed results of patients suffering from co-infections rather than Lyme itself.

11 Where In the World Is Lyme?

In the Caribbean, dogs tested positive for Lyme on supposedly Lyme-free islands. They also tested positive for the co-infections. At this point, it's worth looking at where Lyme is found in the rest of the world. Is there a Lyme-free vacation spot short of the arctic?

If we look at the CDC's map of Lyme, it presents as a progressively advancing army of black dots in the U.S., extending its reach year by year. Very intimidating, and very wrong.

Lyme isn't limited to the areas that the CDC has marked on a map of the U.S. It isn't even limited to the temperate regions that grow the only ticks that the CDC claims can transmit the disease. By 1989 in the U.S., Lyme had been reported in 31 different states, though it's much more common in a few.[xliii]

Once you leave the U.S., it's amazing where you find Lyme. It's all over Europe, but here in the U.S. we rarely hear about

European Lyme. About a third of Germans in one study tested positive for Lyme even back in 1985.[xliv] Other researchers estimated that about 15% of rural Germans had antibodies to Lyme.[xlv] This ongoing level of exposure continued despite another German study that the chances of getting Lyme from a tick bite were only about 4%.[xlvi] Oh, and the complete absence in Europe of the one tick the CDC says is the only tick that transmits Lyme.

In Austria, 4% of bitten soldiers developed a rash, but 20% developed antibodies to Lyme. In Belgium, 10% of the ticks tested positive for Lyme.[xlvii] 86% of deer tested positive for Lyme antibodies in the UK and Ireland.[xlviii] In Sweden, endemic areas had one in four people positive for Lyme, while among city dwellers one in ten were positive for Lyme.[xlix]

On Aland, a Finnish island which is about as far off the beaten track as you can get in Europe, there were seventeen confirmed cases of Lyme.[l] So nowhere in Europe is Lyme-free.

But Lyme isn't limited to the U.S. and Europe. In northern China, doctors estimated about 8% of tick bites resulted in symptoms.[li] Another area of China found 46% of ticks were positive and about 18% of the population had antibodies to Lyme.[lii] In Japan, Lyme cases were found on all its islands.[liii]

And Lyme isn't limited to the temperate zones anywhere on the planet. Remember, we started this journey in the now Lyme positive Caribbean. In Egypt, half a world away, doctors found both animals and humans testing positive for Lyme.[liv]

It can be terrifying to realize that avoiding the climate and the feeding grounds of one tick species isn't going to protect us from Lyme. But the underlying message should be reassuring. Lyme isn't a New England disease or a U.S. disease. It isn't a recent disease. It is an endemic, global illness that has been around for a very, very long time (remember Ötzi).

Even more reassuring is that the dog wisdom model does seem to hold true worldwide. Most people infected with Lyme show no symptoms.

12 Avoiding Lyme

If you believe the CDC, getting Lyme takes a lot of work. Ticks will only bite you if you fail to use simple precautions. Long pants and tick spray are all you need to go hunting or hike safely.

If you're bitten, the CDC says you need worry only if you're bitten by a deer tick, not any other kind of tick. The deer tick needs to be infected with Lyme. You need to leave the tick on your body, unnoticed, for almost two days. Only after all that do you have a chance of getting Lyme, and it's still well below a five percent risk. But if you notice that tick anytime in the first two days and remove it, you won't get Lyme even if it was an infected tick. Just in case, people bitten by documented deer ticks can get a single day's worth of doxycycline, which is more than enough to kill off any Lyme that happened to make it into you.

Getting Lyme: The CDC Recipe

Find a deer tick (Ixodes scapularis only, please).

Make sure it's infected with Lyme properly.

Apply to unprotected skin.

Leave on for at least two days.

Only a tiny chance of Lyme (5%, tops).

Cure: one day of doxycycline antibiotics.

For ILADS, getting Lyme is much, much easier. The tick doesn't have to be a deer tick, it doesn't have to stay on for three days. If you get bitten by any infected tick, for any length of time, you can get Lyme. Once you've gotten Lyme, it never really goes away. It can rear its head any time in the next few years. Your immune system can let it grow slowly inside you. ILADS doctors believe that Lyme can be passed sexually between partners and from mothers to unborn babies. Some ILADS folks even say that Lyme can be passed by saliva, from animals nibbling on your vegetables (or living in your home and licking your face). There is some evidence that Lyme could be passed by urine.[lv]

Getting Lyme: The ILADS Recipe

Just live in an endemic area, you'll probably get it.

Get bitten by any tick.

Or have sex with someone who was.

Or live near animals who might drool on you.

Or eat vegetables that have been licked or urinated on by animals with Lyme

Cure: You wish. Not going to happen.

Treatment: A lifetime supply of antibiotics.

We'd all like to think that the CDC is right, and that ILADS is wrong. Let's look at the first part, that using insecticide will protect you from being bitten. Unfortunately, researchers completely covered in chemically treated clothing that should have protected them got bitten. They did do silly things like sit on fallen logs and lie down in dead leaves. But it turns out some ticks will bite you even if they die in the process.[lvi] So much for just protecting yourself.

13 Treating Lyme

Once you've understood that Lyme is likely worldwide and pretty hard to avoid, treatment seems like a good thing to have on hand. It can even feel like we should all be taking antibiotics all the time. So let's look at the most common treatments.

Doxycycline

Doxycycline is not an inert drug. It can cause diarrhea, photophobia, let your skin burn, and wipe out your good gut bugs so you are more prone to lots of other infectious growths. But it is the mainstay of Lyme treatment. In an endemic area, someone who has been bitten should at least know how they react to doxycycline. Some patients are unaffected, while others simply can't do "doxy" because of the side effects. Many patients wish they'd known that before they came down with advanced Lyme.

At this point most ILADS doctors have moved on from doxycycline alone to a combination of different drugs together.[lvii]

Amoxicillin

In some studies, amoxicillin works as well at killing Lyme as doxycycline. The ILADS doctors say it doesn't kill the Lyme bug, just causes the bug to "spore up" or slow its growth to avoid being killed off. But children who got bitten were given amoxicillin. They seemed to get better, so we're either curing them (CDC docs) or masking a chronic infection (ILADS). In one ILADS test tube study amoxicillin worked as well as doxycycline, and none of the treatments were effective at wiping out Lyme entirely.[lviii] In a Mainer's terms, no matter what drugs you used if you're looking for a Lyme cure, "yah cain't get theah from heah." There's no foolproof combination.

IV Antibiotics

Some ILADS docs want to go directly to IV antibiotics, pumping them directly into the bloodstream. The idea is that you can give a lot more antibiotics a lot quicker, and if you think more is better, then IV is the way to go. I'm sure those using the IV antibiotics can point to numerous cases that got better on IV. But the big studies of IV versus oral doxycycline show it doesn't make much difference in recovery time or cure rate. On the other hand, if my child or loved one had brain symptoms from Lyme I'd probably want IV antibiotics.

Flagyl

Flagyl is an anti-parasitic. It's truly nasty, and can be the worst experience a patient ever has with a drug. Flagyl is given by ILADS doctors in the hope that the spore form of Lyme is wiped out. There are no studies in humans that show that this happens, but again, I'm sure individual patients have been improved by taking Flagyl.

Others (Many Others)

Other medications are also given. Many of them. None of them have any large studies to support their use for Lyme. So yes, your ILADS doctor means well. Yes, he or she has seen great results. But no, that drug is not FDA approved for treating Lyme. So every patient needs to make a medical decision about his or her own care. For each person there is a side effect level, a financial burden level, and a hassle level that ultimately will determine how much treatment he or she will tolerate. It can be very helpful to have these limits clear as you start aggressive treatment.

14 Antibiotic Resistant Lyme?

If Lyme did not gradually develop antibiotic resistance, it would be unlike most other infectious bacteria. One of the things that ILADS doctors don't like to talk about is how dependent on antibiotics they are and how likely it is that Lyme will be completely resistant in our lifetimes.

On the other hand, it must be incredibly reassuring to be a CDC doctor who believes Lyme can be completely cured 100% of the time by just doxycycline.

Early cases, back when Lyme was still erythema chronica migrans, responded well to any antibiotic. Anything would work, penicillin, anything you had on hand. But the honeymoon couldn't last. By the late 1980's doctors in Germany reported Lyme resistance to high dose IV penicillin.[lix] They also found Lyme beginning to be resistant to tetracycline.[lx]

By 1992, researchers documented the beginning of resistance

to doxycycline.[lxi] At this point for Lyme, Azithromycin may slightly outperform doxycycline.[lxii]

Is Lyme performing some ninja level mutation to avoid being killed by antibiotics? Maybe. Lyme shows at least the development of antibiotic tolerance, slowing its growth cycle to accommodate for antibiotics.[lxiii] In a test tube, Lyme shows all sorts of resistance, but CDC doctors are quick to point out that a test tube is different from a human body.[lxiv] A recent monkey study showed a small amount of resistant Lyme still present after antibiotic treatment, which is consistent with what researchers found in Caribbean dogs.[lxv] But CDC docs fired back that the study wasn't valid.[lxvi] Meanwhile German doctors have documented the failure of all forms of antibiotics for some cases of Lyme.[lxvii]

At this point, ILADS doctors have moved well beyond antibiotics to anti-cancer medications and antibiotics repeated in pulsed doses over and over. These methods may work in a test tube, but they have not been studied in human trials.[lxviii] At the same time, other researchers testing for Lyme weaknesses have found over a hundred currently unused drugs that block Lyme in a test tube.[lxix] So we'll likely see new combinations from the ILADS doctors in the near future.

15 Is Lyme Autoimmune?

Yes, Lyme is an infectious illness. But are the symptoms of Lyme due to the infection or the immune system's overreaction? Currently our treatments are based on wiping out the infection, but perhaps at some point we should focus on calming an overactive immune system as well.

Even the original rash from Lyme has an immune basis. The Lyme bacteria triggers the immune system, and the immune system's response triggers the rash.[lxx] In the absence of the Lyme bacteria, researchers can cause the same rash just by injected animals with drugs that mimic the immune system's chemical response.[lxxi] In other words, you don't need to be exposed to actual Lyme to get the most distinctive of Lyme symptom. Your immune system can do it for you.

One of the most dramatic side effects of Lyme in Connecticut was the appearance of arthritic symptoms. In one study, out of thirty-two people with Lyme, twenty-four had the classic rash, and nineteen developed arthritis. But the arthritis could be delayed, with as much as twenty weeks between bite and the beginning of pain. If half of those getting Lyme develop arthritis, then something dramatic is taking place in the immune system. Many of those patients recovered (without or without antibiotics) but some of them continued to have arthritic symptoms for months afterward.[lxxii]

Another study at the same time calculated that as many as one in ten affected Lyme children would be struck by arthritic symptoms.[lxxiii] It was the arthritis, not the rash, that brought the international medical attention to Lyme.

Tracking untreated Lyme over six years in adults, researchers found that by two years out more than half of the untreated adults had experienced at least one arthritic flare up from Lyme. These decreased in frequency over the next four years, but about ten percent of untreated patients had permanent arthritis.[lxxiv]

As early as 1987 researchers found some Lyme patients had positive rheumatoid factor (similar to what is found in rheumatoid arthritis), showing that their bodies were attacking themselves.[lxxv] The early studies of Lyme found immune cells in the arthritic joints. These immune cells become irreversible solids at low temperatures (cryoglobulins), and gunked up the joint long after the active Lyme infection was resolved. All the Lyme patients who continued to have arthritic symptoms also continued to have these immune cells in their joints.[lxxvi] But in some unlucky Lyme patients, these immune cells remained throughout the body, leading to all sorts of other symptoms.[lxxvii]

So the answer for these patients might be lots of antibiotics initially to avoid the autoimmune response. But antibiotics wouldn't resolve the later symptoms. For those, doctors might need to switch to treating patients for autoimmune disease.

It's not just that the long term antibiotics might not help. They might even make things worse. The "Herxheimer reaction" is an autoimmune response to taking antibiotics, which is seen as a good thing in the doctors using aggressive antibiotic treatments. As the spirochetes die off, ILADS doctors believe that a good immune system will mount a strong defense. Usually it produces fever for a few hours, but the Herxheimer reactions can also include: contractions in pregnancy, worsening liver and kidney function, difficulty breathing, heart injury, low blood pressure, brain inflammation, alterations in consciousness, seizures, and strokes.[lxxviii] If that sounds like the healing reaction could be worse than the disease, that's right.

Rather than trying to force their way through a reaction, patients would be better served to go slower with their antibiotics, allowing the body time to process and heal. Any ILADS doctor who tells you that a stroke is an acceptable side effect from a "healing reaction" has lost perspective. And any ILADS doctor worth their salt knows that antibiotics, no matter how powerful, won't kill all the Lyme bacteria.[lxxix] But at this point most ILADS doctors still are not moving from the infectious model to treating Chronic Lyme as at least partially an autoimmune disease. Just as the CDC doesn't acknowledge that Chronic Lyme exists, ILADS doctors have trouble thinking that it might not be infectious Lyme after all.

16 Does Chronic Lyme Exist? Yes And No.

Whether you call it Chronic Lyme, Post-Lyme Disease Syndrome, or the Canadian Alternatively Diagnosed Chronic Lyme Syndrome, something is going on in these patients. While we now know what caused the disease in Lyme, Connecticut, that hasn't made the situation for sufferers that much better. Some of the people infected by that 1975 outbreak still think they have the symptoms of Lyme.[lxxx]

If we try to find a middle ground, both the CDC and ILADS agree that untreated Lyme can cause chronic symptoms. ILADS goes further and says that co-infections cause many problems in patients. The CDC has trouble acknowledging that co-infections are major problem, but they would say that an untreated co-infection could cause symptoms. Given how many co-infections there are, (the list is ten plus and growing) isn't it possible that some of the people who experience ongoing symptoms of Lyme are really experiencing another illness, a co-infection that hasn't been properly treated?

Both the CDC and ILADS also like to ignore that the tests they're using aren't that accurate, with the best lab test results catching about 80% of Lyme.[lxxxi] Doing multiple tests can increase accuracy, but that accuracy can still depend on how long it has been since the tick bite. Patients who have previously been bitten may also show up positive in future tests without a new bite.[lxxxii] So even ILADS doctors could be treating the wrong infection if a patient tests positive for a past infection with Lyme and doesn't want to pay the extra money for co-infection testing (which isn't much more accurate, and may be less so).

Shouldn't there be a middle ground here? Some people might be positive for Lyme but have symptoms that have nothing to do with Lyme. Other people could test negative for Lyme but still have symptoms from the disease or a co-infection. We know that other medical lab tests have both false positives and false negatives, and that lab results are not the final word on a diagnosis.

But with Lyme, the lab results can determine insurance coverage for treatment. It can also determine if patients receive antibiotics or antipsychotics. And that means it matters a great deal how a patient is initially diagnosed and by whom.

Despite the controversy between CDC labs and IgenX, both labs come back with similar results (three positive markers, five positive markers, etc.). But they are interpreted entirely differently by the doctors receiving the tests.[lxxxiii] Basing treatment entirely on doctors' preferences makes the whole process of diagnosing and treating Lyme wildly subjective and all over the map. Visit a CDC practitioner, test negative (according to his lab interpretation) and get sent home with nothing. Visit an ILADS practitioner, test positive (according to his lab interpretation) and get a chemical cocktail more potent than anything else you may have ever taken in your life. That cocktail needs to be followed for months with no promise of success. But many people feel like they have no other options.[lxxxiv]

And then we have states where Lyme disease is endemic. That means whatever treatment or non-treatment you receive may need to be done again and again because you get rebitten by ticks. These states have become more numerous and far-reaching in the last few decades. What is a person to do, besides stop having pets and doing a tick check every twenty minutes even though they now live in a bubble and never go outside out of fear?

To really find an answer to Chronic Lyme, we should go back. Not to the good old days before Lyme, but to that confused, frightening time between when Lyme was first seen as a disease and before it was documented to come only from one species of Lyme tick with a very specific area of transmission.

Before We "Knew Everything" About Lyme

When Lyme was first recognized, the Europeans were caught off guard. They didn't immediately think that Lyme was endemic in their countries, but once they started looking British, Scandinavian and German medical journals all reported cases of Lyme.[lxxxv] Looking back, U.S. soldiers returning from Europe were catching Lyme and bringing it back with them.[lxxxvi] But since Europe had none of the same ticks as the U.S., they documented that other ticks could carry the infection in Europe.[lxxxvii] Some of the researchers tested birds because they suspected the Lyme cases were somehow brought over from the U.S. and found that the birds could harbor Lyme.[lxxxviii] More recently, the U.S. has confirmed that migrating birds are positive for Lyme.[lxxxix]

In the U.S., Lyme was found almost simultaneously in three different areas: the northeastern U.S., Wisconsin, and on the west coast. In two of the areas the "right" tick was present, but the west coast Lyme clearly involved a different tick.[xc] So when Lyme was first documented transmission was reported by multiple ticks, and there were even reports of possible mosquito or flea transmission.[xci] The west coast cases of Lyme symptoms were particularly bad and clearly not transmitted by the same tick as in the northeast.

Now well-documented cases have occurred in the south of the U.S., caused by another tick, and CDC experts have decided to call it Southern Tick Associated Rash Illness (STARI) despite the fact that, "(S)ymptoms of STARI are similar to early Lyme."[xcii] That's just what the Lyme Wars need, another distinct illness that looks like Lyme, is transmitted like Lyme, but officially isn't Lyme. The CDC just decided to define it as something else.

So whether Chronic Lyme disease exists may be simply a matter of definition.

If you define Lyme as an active, long-term infection by a single distinct species of the Lyme bacteria, transmitted by only one kind of tick, it probably doesn't exist. Older texts list at least sixteen species of Lyme bacteria[xciii] from all over the world[xciv] and the Mayo Clinic recently announced the discovery of a new species of Lyme bacteria.[xcv] But older CDC doctors very narrowly defining Lyme to one bacteria, with ongoing active infection, and passed by one tick may be right that Chronic Lyme doesn't exist.

The definition may be technically, academically correct. But that definition doesn't account for different species of Lyme bacteria, co-infections, different ticks transmitting the bacteria, or any kind of autoimmune response to the tick bites that continues after the infection is gone. When these "not strictly just active

Lyme passed by one tick" cases are taken into account, then Chronic Lyme very broadly defined certainly occurs in many patients.

On one side we have the strict definition, one that requires the exclusion of different species of Lyme, co-infections, or an autoimmune response. On the other side we have a very broad definition that includes different ticks, different species of Lyme, and the co-infections.

Both definitions may be correct, in the same way that someone is correct when they say they have the "'flu." What they have may not strictly be influenza as documented by the CDC, which only lists one set of viruses as being influenza. But we would all acknowledge they are probably not "making up" their symptoms of illness. They likely have something similar enough to be treated and acknowledged to be "flu-like" enough to justify medical treatment and necessary time off from work. Even the CDC has expanded its own definition of death from influenza to include patients who died of pneumonia after previously having the influenza virus. They didn't die of influenza, but we all agree that influenza was a likely cause or partial cause of their deaths.

For CDC doctors, Chronic Lyme may not be a reality, because they cannot find an active infection over an extended time from the one species of Lyme bacteria they recognize as the only true Lyme. For ILADS doctors with a much broader definition of Lyme,

Chronic Lyme always exists when symptoms occur because they are always on the brink of finding a new species of Lyme bacteria or a new co-infection. So when both sides scream at each other, they are not guilty of lying or denying the facts, only of not listening to the definition of Chronic Lyme made by the other side.

17 Will We Get a Human Vaccine?

We already had one. It failed to provide long term immunity.[xcvi] So patients had to get annual shots. The side effects from the vaccine included arthritis-like symptoms, leading to class-action lawsuits. Getting the vaccine led to testing false-positive on Lyme labs for the disease, making it hard to tell how well the vaccine was working.[xcvii] Ultimately, the vaccine went off the market due to poor sales.

At this point, researchers recognize that we need a new vaccine, but it needs to address a range of different species of Lyme, as well as the co-infections. That's a high bar to climb, especially if you're a vaccine manufacturer looking at previous class action lawsuits if you screw up. So there may be a vaccine, but not very soon.[xcviii]

Dogs do have a vaccine. It has to be done annually like a flu shot. Swelling of the site can last as long as a week.[xcix] And some dogs still get Lyme despite the shot.[c] But it does drop the infection rate by about 80%, which is comparable to some human vaccines for other diseases currently on the market.

18 Other Treatments

Now we get into the wild and wooly world of alternative medicine. We've got herbs, physical treatments, light, sound, energetic healing, homeopathics, and patent Chinese formulas. Do they work? We don't know. None of them have any studies behind them. The CDC is happy to tell you so, as well as list all the treatments that don't work and are just going to rip you off.[ci]

At the same time, ILADS labs are testing various substances in combination with doxycycline, and show that a number of different compounds help doxycycline kill Lyme in test tube studies.[cii]

A few of these compounds that help kill Lyme may seem familiar: rosemary, Vitamin D, and Vitamin C. Also kelp.[ciii] Why aren't these aren't being used more in treatment by both CDC and ILADS docs? Because the focus is almost entirely on antibiotic or other drug regimens.

What about other common alternative treatments? How many good quality studies have been done on Lyme and acupuncture, chiropractic, naturopathy, homeopathy, massage, herbs, or probiotics? None. No one has moved beyond arguing over how many drugs to give patients. Both sides agree that patients may have symptoms that continue after antibiotic treatment, although they don't agree on why those symptoms continue. But that hasn't yet reached a point where either side is seriously pursuing research on other treatments. A preliminary study of things like massage for Lyme shows it might be as useful for long-term pain as another round of antibiotics.[civ]

For those wretched folks post-Lyme treatment with continuing symptoms, my apologies. The medical profession has done a terrible job of putting patients first and egos last when working with Lyme. If you want to get rid of your Lyme biofilms, you could take months of antibiotics, or you could switch sweeteners. Stevia showed the same effect (in a test tube) as doxycycline in breaking down resistant Lyme.[cv]

19 Living With Lyme

How likely are we to get Lyme? In an endemic state, it's a real possibility. How likely? We don't know. Even during the original Lyme outbreak, people were thirty times more likely to get Lyme on one side of the river in Lyme, Connecticut than on the other side.[cvi]

But at least when we get bitten we have immunity? Not if we're like mice, who only mount an immune response to Lyme of less than a year.[cvii] In comparison, human patients who have untreated Lyme may never have a normal immune response to Lyme even if they've been treated. Their antibodies drop, but never all the way down to a normal level.[cviii] So if you suffer for Lyme a while, you do have at least semi-permanent immunity. That may or may not be a good thing, depending on how much of the symptoms of Lyme are actually autoimmune.

Surely after decades we have long-term follow-up studies on patients treated for Lyme? In New York, men and women with Lyme followed for twenty years showed no differences in any area except that women came in for follow-up much more frequently.[cix] About ten percent of those followed continued to have Chronic Lyme/Post-Lyme Syndrome symptoms, but after about twenty years only about five percent still had symptoms and none of them experienced any impairment from the symptoms.[cx]

After being followed for years from an initial case in 1962, one in five residents of Great Island, Massachusetts eventually developed Lyme. Of those who didn't get any Lyme symptoms, about one in ten had antibodies to Lyme that lasted for years.[cxi] So at least in those communities some people had antibodies showing possible ongoing exposure without symptoms. Other studies have shown a similar pattern of symptoms and antibodies, with the range of those with symptoms around ten percent.[cxii]

A Lyme Diet and Lifestyle?

For those of us who clearly live in an endemic state, is there a diet and lifestyle we should follow besides the obvious, "Don't get bit?" Out of over twelve thousand articles on Lyme, exactly ten mention diet and twenty-five mention exercise.

If we were mice, we'd have a pretty good idea of what not to eat. The standard American, high-fat diet worked directly with the Lyme to suppress the immune systems - of mice.[cxiii] Adding fish to a mouse diet didn't seem to decrease inflammation.[cxiv] Human results may vary.

Our exercise routine perhaps should mimic the low impact aerobic workouts that the CDC docs recommend for Chronic Lyme sufferers.[cxv]

Beyond that, we have only speculation. We do know that the Lyme bacteria likes to eat very specific foods: sugars. These are usually available in our bloodstream, but having a ton of extra sugar won't help us and might help Lyme grow.[cxvi]

Lyme upsets the immune system, generating inflammation.[cxvii] Something as simple as sufficient vitamin D may decrease that inflammation by more than half.[cxviii]

If we look at Lyme symptoms as being at least partly autoimmune, then our path toward health is clearer. All of the things we would do to care for a cold would apply: getting enough rest, fluids, eating correctly, avoiding excess stresses, dressing warmly, nurturing ourselves generally. It's heartening to think that these same habits could prevent or lessen the effects of Lyme.

20 A Different Discussion

So, what is a patient to do? How do you find your way through Lyme to treatment, and how worried should you be about Lyme if you don't have it (or just think you don't have it) yet?

Let me say that both sides are right. The CDC docs are right that way too many people are being diagnosed with Lyme who have something else, even if that something else is a co-infection. Before you go down the Lyme path, first see if you have anything else. Treating for Lyme is very time intensive if you follow the ILADS docs' plans. If the mixed drug cocktails of the ILADS docs don't solve your problems, you may end up poorer, sicker, and now without hope because you've got Chronic Lyme eating at you.

But the ILADS docs have some really good arguments in favor of treatment. Not all the patients they treat have Lyme, but many improve on their cocktails and wider lifestyle treatments. At some point ILADS docs stop treating the Lyme and start treating the whole person, which is a whole lot more care and sympathy than that person will receive from a CDC doc. Patients do improve under ILADS care for any number of reasons, but likely because the ILADS docs will keep trying things until something works.

And some of the patients do have Chronic Lyme. Yes, even narrowly defined by the CDC as an active infection of the one species. They are extremely rare, but they do exist. It's ridiculous to think that Lyme, of all infectious illnesses, has built up no drug-resistance. It's also ridiculous to claim that every patient will improve on the same short antibiotic treatment. Within their medical studies, CDC docs will talk about giving different drugs when they run into resistance, or more antibiotics if the symptoms continue, but they ignore that medical reality when they make their general guidelines.

So some of you do have Chronic Lyme. Someday (probably when this generation of docs has retired) we may have a consensus that it exists.

But many of you don't have Chronic Lyme, you have something else. Maybe even something that we don't have a name for yet. Whether or not that is best treated using lots of drugs and antibiotics, we don't know.

But what if you don't have any symptoms? That's fine, leave yourself alone. Don't let ILADS docs tell you that your brain is rotting if there is no evidence that it is. In an endemic area (which may well be much of the world) some percentage of people and animals will have antibodies to Lyme. It doesn't mean they have an active infection, and it doesn't mean that they will ever develop an active infection. You may simply be immune, get bitten again, and still be immune. Just because Lyme is scary doesn't make it fundamentally different from any of the other infectious diseases we encounter in our lives.

Should we avoid getting bitten? Absolutely. Can we avoid getting exposed? Not likely. We're surrounded by Lyme, and if you believe the ILADS folks, it's really easy to catch.

Think about Lyme the same way you think about the flu. You don't want to catch it, you try to avoid it. But if and when you get it, you want to treat it as quick as you can and move on with your life once the symptoms drop down. The death rate from Lyme, by the way, is very tiny compared to the death rate from the flu. So it really makes no sense to spend more of your time freaking out about a possible tick exposure when half your coworkers are sneezing on you.

One hopeful thought. The outbreak of Lyme in Connecticut struck primarily the young people. The older people, those who normally have weaker immune systems, had much less illness. So it is very likely that they had already been exposed to Lyme in some way. Our immune system handles a vast array of possible agents, and a little low-grade exposure to Lyme (short tick bite, a dog's lick) may prevent you from getting a huge reaction to it. In other words, living in an endemic area (or an endemic world) may naturally generate some immunity over time.

Remember dog wisdom. A lot of dogs got exposed, only a few got symptoms. Most of them were fine. The most recent estimate of Lyme exposure in the U.S. is based on the idea that about one in ten people will develop symptoms. That's how we went from 30,000 cases to 300,000 exposures.

Yes, we should be cautious. But the Cochrane database estimates the chances of getting Lyme from a tick bite at 2%. If you have a one in ten chance of showing any symptoms, that means any given tick bite is pretty much likely to be harmless. We all know people with Lyme, and with Chronic Lyme symptoms, but the chances are very good for every person with Chronic Lyme there are nine times as many people who've gotten the illness, have antibodies, and may never show any symptoms now or in the future.

So be careful out there, but don't be paranoid. Hopefully if you do get bitten and need help, you now understand who to go to for the help you want. You also understand why some of your doctors believe you and others don't. For those of you who need a short checklist, here are the steps I would do for my family in the case of a tick bite.

Tick bite plan (for my family)

Identify tick (most are big, mottled dog ticks)

Watch bite location and monitor symptoms

Go to regular doctor if there are symptoms, get CDC test.

If the test is negative and symptoms go away, let it go.

If the test is negative and symptoms continue,

consider other possible diagnoses.

Visit an ILADS doctor. Go over treatment plan.

Visit a second ILADS doctor, compare plans.

Commit to three to six months of plan.

Reconsider at one, three, and six months.

I encourage every family to come up with their own plan. It's a little like fire safety, you never want to put your plan into action. But you want to be prepared. The last thing you want to do is ignore a fire (CDC) or use a fire hose on a tiny smolder (ILADS). We can't fix the Lyme Wars, but we can find the middle ground for our own loved ones.

ABOUT THE AUTHOR

Dr. Christopher Maloney, N.D. went to Swarthmore College, got his premedical diploma at Harvard University, and his medical degree from the National University of Natural Medicine. He does not belong to ILADS or the CDC, but he knows and loves smart doctors who belong to both groups. His dream is to be able to have them both over to dinner without having to hide the knives and forks before they arrive.

If you enjoyed this book, please review it online. In today's marketplace of ideas your opinion matters.

Other books from Dr. Maloney can be found on Amazon. He has written about the gut microbiome, NF1, colon cancer, and Zika.

Endnotes

These have been simplified for patient use. Signing on to pubmed from any library computer and putting in the number of the abstract or article will give you the ability to do your own research and come to your own conclusions.

i https://www.ncbi.nlm.nih.gov/pubmed/1790102
ii https://www.ncbi.nlm.nih.gov/pubmed/3885366
iii https://www.ncbi.nlm.nih.gov/pubmed/826813
iv http://news.nationalgeographic.com/news/2013/10/131016-otzi-ice-man-mummy-five-facts/
v http://www.ct.gov/dph/lib/dph/infectious_diseases/lyme/1976_circular_letter.pdf
vi https://www.ncbi.nlm.nih.gov/pubmed/658948
vii http://www.nytimes.com/2004/02/15/nyregion/heaping-more-dirt-on-plum-i.html?_r=0
viii https://www.ncbi.nlm.nih.gov/pmc/articles/PMC4443866/
ix https://www.ncbi.nlm.nih.gov/pubmed/25451629
x https://www.ncbi.nlm.nih.gov/pubmed/25999221
xi https://www.scientificamerican.com/article/new-cause-for-lyme-disease-complicates-already-murky-diagnosis1/
xii https://www.ncbi.nlm.nih.gov/pubmed/2683415
xiii https://www.cdc.gov/lyme/treatment/prolonged/index.html
xiv https://www.ncbi.nlm.nih.gov/pubmed/19013025
xv http://ilads.org/lyme/getlymesmart.pdf
xvi https://www.ncbi.nlm.nih.gov/pmc/articles/PMC3636972/
xvii https://www.ncbi.nlm.nih.gov/pubmed/1980573
xviii https://www.ncbi.nlm.nih.gov/pubmed/8506882
xix https://www.ncbi.nlm.nih.gov/pubmed/4013743
xx https://www.ncbi.nlm.nih.gov/pubmed/2346158
xxi https://www.ncbi.nlm.nih.gov/pmc/articles/PMC2901226/
xxii https://www.cdc.gov/rmsf/doxycycline/
xxiii https://www.ncbi.nlm.nih.gov/pubmed/19711595
xxiv https://www.ncbi.nlm.nih.gov/pubmed/2346158
xxv https://www.ncbi.nlm.nih.gov/pmc/articles/PMC3540629/
xxvi https://www.ncbi.nlm.nih.gov/pubmed/26082507
xxvii http://www.nejm.org/doi/full/10.1056/NEJMra072023
xxviii http://www.igenex.com/Website/why-igenex/comprehensive-testing/
xxix https://www.ncbi.nlm.nih.gov/pubmed/24794819
xxx https://www.ncbi.nlm.nih.gov/pubmed/20382722
xxxi https://www.ncbi.nlm.nih.gov/pubmed/27931077
xxxii https://www.ncbi.nlm.nih.gov/pubmed/27686962
xxxiii https://www.ncbi.nlm.nih.gov/pubmed/26607686
xxxiv https://www.ncbi.nlm.nih.gov/pubmed/27013465

[xxxv] https://www.ncbi.nlm.nih.gov/pubmed/26459093
[xxxvi] https://www.nimh.nih.gov/health/statistics/prevalence/any-mental-illness-ami-among-us-adults.shtml
[xxxvii] https://www.ncbi.nlm.nih.gov/pubmed/25325316
[xxxviii] https://www.ncbi.nlm.nih.gov/pubmed/23335965
[xxxix] https://www.ncbi.nlm.nih.gov/pubmed/23335965
[xl] https://www.ncbi.nlm.nih.gov/pubmed/4013743
[xli] https://www.ncbi.nlm.nih.gov/pubmed/19017912
[xlii] https://www.ncbi.nlm.nih.gov/pubmed/23885337
[xliii] https://www.ncbi.nlm.nih.gov/pubmed/2682955
[xliv] https://www.ncbi.nlm.nih.gov/pubmed/3905325
[xlv] https://www.ncbi.nlm.nih.gov/pubmed/3591095
[xlvi] https://www.ncbi.nlm.nih.gov/pubmed/3591103
[xlvii] https://www.ncbi.nlm.nih.gov/pubmed/2683538
[xlviii] https://www.ncbi.nlm.nih.gov/pubmed/2880076
[xlix] https://www.ncbi.nlm.nih.gov/pubmed/2371545
[l] https://www.ncbi.nlm.nih.gov/pubmed/2320965
[li] https://www.ncbi.nlm.nih.gov/pubmed/3190101
[lii] https://www.ncbi.nlm.nih.gov/pubmed/2065539
[liii] https://www.ncbi.nlm.nih.gov/pubmed/1885848
[liv] https://www.ncbi.nlm.nih.gov/pubmed/25239124
[lv] https://www.ncbi.nlm.nih.gov/pubmed/17225014
[lvi] https://www.ncbi.nlm.nih.gov/pubmed/15061284
[lvii] https://www.ncbi.nlm.nih.gov/pubmed/27242757
[lviii] https://www.ncbi.nlm.nih.gov/pubmed/21753890
[lix] https://www.ncbi.nlm.nih.gov/pubmed/3702279
[lx] https://www.ncbi.nlm.nih.gov/pubmed/3580012
[lxi] https://www.ncbi.nlm.nih.gov/pubmed/1337070
[lxii] https://www.ncbi.nlm.nih.gov/pubmed/8387966
[lxiii] https://www.ncbi.nlm.nih.gov/pmc/articles/PMC4594320/
[lxiv] https://www.ncbi.nlm.nih.gov/pubmed/26014929
[lxv] https://www.ncbi.nlm.nih.gov/pubmed/22253822
[lxvi] https://www.ncbi.nlm.nih.gov/pubmed/22620495
[lxvii] https://www.ncbi.nlm.nih.gov/pubmed/16530006
[lxviii] https://www.ncbi.nlm.nih.gov/pubmed/26014929
[lxix] https://www.ncbi.nlm.nih.gov/pmc/articles/PMC4827596/#SD1-dddt-10-1307
[lxx] https://www.ncbi.nlm.nih.gov/pubmed/3577475
[lxxi] https://www.ncbi.nlm.nih.gov/pubmed/3495083
[lxxii] https://www.ncbi.nlm.nih.gov/pubmed/869348
[lxxiii] https://www.ncbi.nlm.nih.gov/pubmed/836338
[lxxiv] https://www.ncbi.nlm.nih.gov/pubmed/3662285

lxxv https://www.ncbi.nlm.nih.gov/pubmed/3668982
lxxvi https://www.ncbi.nlm.nih.gov/pubmed/109097
lxxvii https://www.ncbi.nlm.nih.gov/pubmed/503166
lxxviii https://www.ncbi.nlm.nih.gov/pubmed/28077740
lxxix https://www.ncbi.nlm.nih.gov/pubmed/21753890
lxxx http://news.nationalgeographic.com/news/2014/02/140228-lyme-disease-borrelia-burgdorferi-deer-tick-science
lxxxi https://www.ncbi.nlm.nih.gov/pubmed/27920571
lxxxii https://www.ncbi.nlm.nih.gov/pmc/articles/PMC4918152/
lxxxiii https://www.ncbi.nlm.nih.gov/pubmed/25182244/
lxxxiv http://www.newyorker.com/magazine/2013/07/01/the-lyme-wars
lxxxv https://www.ncbi.nlm.nih.gov/pmc/articles/PMC1608178/?page=1
lxxxvi https://www.ncbi.nlm.nih.gov/pubmed/730458
lxxxvii https://www.ncbi.nlm.nih.gov/pubmed/6839977
lxxxviii https://www.ncbi.nlm.nih.gov/pubmed/6516460
lxxxix https://www.ncbi.nlm.nih.gov/pubmed/19198527
xc https://www.ncbi.nlm.nih.gov/pubmed/496106
xci https://www.ncbi.nlm.nih.gov/pubmed/6516458, https://www.ncbi.nlm.nih.gov/pubmed/4075471, https://www.ncbi.nlm.nih.gov/pubmed/3542350
xcii https://www.ncbi.nlm.nih.gov/pubmed/19522220
xciii https://www.ncbi.nlm.nih.gov/pmc/articles/PMC373079/?page=2
xciv https://www.ncbi.nlm.nih.gov/pubmed/21414082
xcv https://www.cdc.gov/media/releases/2016/p0208-lyme-disease.html
xcvi https://www.cdc.gov/lyme/prev/vaccine.html
xcvii https://www.ncbi.nlm.nih.gov/pubmed/10617720
xcviii https://www.ncbi.nlm.nih.gov/pmc/articles/PMC3569838/
xcix https://www.ncbi.nlm.nih.gov/pubmed/9004447
c https://www.ncbi.nlm.nih.gov/pubmed/8320151
ci https://www.ncbi.nlm.nih.gov/pubmed/25852124
cii https://www.ncbi.nlm.nih.gov/pubmed/27570483
ciii https://www.ncbi.nlm.nih.gov/pubmed/26457476
civ https://www.ncbi.nlm.nih.gov/pubmed/23429967
cv https://www.ncbi.nlm.nih.gov/pubmed/26716015
cvi https://www.ncbi.nlm.nih.gov/pubmed/727200
cvii https://www.ncbi.nlm.nih.gov/pubmed/9317005
cviii https://www.ncbi.nlm.nih.gov/pubmed/7884218
cix https://www.ncbi.nlm.nih.gov/pubmed/27230991
cx https://www.ncbi.nlm.nih.gov/pubmed/26385994
cxi https://www.ncbi.nlm.nih.gov/pubmed/3722867
cxii https://www.ncbi.nlm.nih.gov/pmc/articles/PMC4657537/
cxiii https://www.ncbi.nlm.nih.gov/pubmed/27794208

cxiv https://www.ncbi.nlm.nih.gov/pubmed/22695969
cxv https://www.ncbi.nlm.nih.gov/pubmed/27922168
cxvi https://www.ncbi.nlm.nih.gov/pubmed/15668016
cxvii https://www.ncbi.nlm.nih.gov/pubmed/23024745
cxviii https://www.ncbi.nlm.nih.gov/pubmed/20691220

www.ingramcontent.com/pod-product-compliance
Lightning Source LLC
Chambersburg PA
CBHW071244170526
45165CB00003B/1236